GALLBLADDER DISEASE

Commonly Due to Gallstones

Complete Guide to Understanding and Managing Gallbladder Disease and Gallstones with Dietary Adjustments, Treatment Options, and Surgical Interventions

Cormac Cristiano

Disclaimer

The information provided in *Gallbladder Disease – Commonly Due to Gallstones: Complete Guide to Understanding and Managing Gallbladder Disease and Gallstones with Dietary Adjustments, Treatment Options, and Surgical Interventions* is intended for educational and informational purposes only. This book does not serve as a substitute for professional medical advice, diagnosis, or treatment. Always consult with a qualified healthcare provider regarding any questions or concerns you may have about gallbladder disease, gallstones, or other medical conditions.

The author and publisher have made every effort to ensure the accuracy and completeness of the information presented in this book. However, they do not assume any liability for any errors or omissions or for any consequences resulting from the application of the information contained herein.

Reliance on any information provided in this book is solely at your own risk.

Furthermore, the author and publisher do not endorse, recommend, or have any affiliation with any specific individual, product, website, organization, or other entities that may be referenced or mentioned within this book. All references and mentions are provided strictly for informational purposes only and do not constitute endorsement or approval.

If you suspect you have a medical problem, please seek prompt medical attention. Never disregard or delay professional medical advice based on information from this book.

About This Book

The book "Gallbladder Disease – Commonly Due to Gallstones: Complete Guide to Understanding and Managing Gallbladder Disease and Gallstones with Dietary Adjustments, Treatment Options, and Surgical Interventions" serves as an invaluable resource for individuals seeking to comprehend the complexities of gallbladder disease, particularly those related to gallstones.

This comprehensive guide delves into the vital functions of the gallbladder and highlights the potential health risks posed by gallstones, providing readers with a foundational understanding of how these issues can significantly affect overall health and well-being.

By outlining the essential role the gallbladder plays in digestion and the potential consequences of its dysfunction, the book lays the groundwork for recognizing symptoms early and understanding the importance of timely medical intervention.

A critical aspect of this guide is its thorough examination of gallstones, including their definition, types, and formation mechanisms. It addresses the myriad of risk factors contributing to gallstone development, such as obesity, dietary choices, genetics, and other medical conditions. By exploring these contributing factors, the book empowers readers to make informed lifestyle changes that can significantly mitigate their risk of developing gallbladder disease. Furthermore, it emphasizes the importance of dietary habits and how the foods one consumes can directly influence gallbladder health.

The book also provides detailed insights into the anatomy of the gallbladder, elucidating its structure, function, and relation to surrounding organs such as the liver and pancreas. This foundational knowledge enhances the reader's appreciation for the gallbladder's role in fat digestion and overall digestive health. It covers common symptoms of gallbladder issues, diagnostic procedures, and the impact of gallbladder disease on daily life, ensuring that readers are well-equipped to recognize and address any health concerns that may arise.

In terms of treatment options, this guide offers a balanced view of both non-surgical and surgical interventions, detailing the significance of dietary modifications as a first-line approach to managing gallbladder disease. Readers will learn about various treatment modalities, including the introduction of laparoscopic cholecystectomy, and gain insights into post-operative care and recovery processes. This information is crucial for anyone facing the prospect of surgery, as it helps demystify the experience and prepares individuals for what lies ahead.

Dietary adjustments play a pivotal role in maintaining gallbladder health, and this guide provides practical advice on what foods to include or avoid to foster a gallbladder-friendly diet. It emphasizes the significance of hydration, fiber intake, and healthy fats while also offering meal planning tips and sample meal ideas. These dietary strategies are not only essential for individuals managing gallbladder disease but can also be beneficial for those looking to prevent its onset.

Moreover, the book addresses the lifestyle changes that can support gallbladder health, such as the importance of regular exercise, stress management, and weight maintenance. By fostering a holistic approach to health, it encourages readers to develop sustainable habits that promote overall well-being.

For those facing surgical interventions, the guide provides a thorough overview of what to expect before, during, and after surgery, as well as the recovery process and long-term effects of living without a gallbladder. This information is critical for alleviating anxieties surrounding surgery and guiding individuals through their recovery journey.

Finally, the book tackles common concerns and frequently asked questions, addressing essential topics such as prevention strategies, managing symptoms, and finding support resources. By fostering an open dialogue about gallbladder disease, it encourages readers to take an active role in their health management and empowers them to seek the information and assistance they need.

Overall, this comprehensive guide serves as an essential tool for anyone looking to understand and manage gallbladder disease and gallstones effectively. With its engaging tone and in-depth exploration of all aspects of gallbladder health, it is a must-have resource for individuals seeking to enhance their quality of life through informed dietary and lifestyle choices.

Table of Contents

Introduction

Overview of Gallbladder Function and Its Importance in Digestion

The gallbladder is a small, pear-shaped organ located beneath the liver, and its primary function is to store and concentrate bile, a digestive fluid produced by the liver. Bile helps break down fats in the small intestine, aiding in nutrient absorption. When you eat a fatty meal, the gallbladder contracts and releases bile into the small intestine, which facilitates the digestion of fats and ensures that your body can utilize essential fatty acids and fat-soluble vitamins effectively.

Understanding the gallbladder's role in digestion highlights the importance of maintaining its health. A well-functioning gallbladder contributes to efficient digestion and nutrient absorption. When problems arise, such as gallbladder disease or gallstones, this process can be disrupted, leading to digestive issues, discomfort, and nutritional deficiencies. Regularly eating a balanced diet can support gallbladder health and prevent potential complications.

Common Causes of Gallbladder Disease, Focusing on Gallstones

Gallbladder disease often results from the formation of gallstones, which are hardened deposits of digestive fluid that can develop in the gallbladder. The most common type of gallstones are cholesterol stones, which occur when there's an imbalance in the substances that make up bile. Risk factors for gallstone formation include obesity, rapid weight loss, pregnancy, and a diet high in fat and cholesterol. To minimize the risk, it's advisable to maintain a healthy weight, eat a balanced diet rich in fiber, and stay hydrated.

Other factors contributing to gallbladder disease include inflammation (cholecystitis), infection, or blockage of the bile ducts. Symptoms may include pain in the upper right abdomen, nausea, and digestive disturbances. Regular check-ups with a healthcare provider can help identify potential gallbladder issues early, allowing for timely dietary and lifestyle adjustments or medical interventions to prevent complications associated with gallstones.

Understanding Gallstones

Definition and Types of Gallstones

Gallstones are hardened deposits that can form in the gallbladder, a small organ beneath the liver responsible for storing bile. There are primarily two types of gallstones: cholesterol gallstones and pigment gallstones. Cholesterol gallstones are yellow-green in color and are primarily made of hardened cholesterol, whereas pigment gallstones are darker and composed of bilirubin, a substance produced from the breakdown of red blood cells.

Understanding the types of gallstones is essential for managing gallbladder disease effectively. Cholesterol gallstones are more common in individuals who are overweight or have a high-cholesterol diet, while pigment gallstones often occur in people with certain medical conditions, such as liver cirrhosis or infections in the biliary tract. Knowing the type can help in choosing the right treatment or dietary changes.

Risk Factors Associated with Gallstone Formation

Several risk factors contribute to the formation of gallstones, including obesity, rapid weight loss, pregnancy, and age. Individuals over 40 years old are at an increased risk, as are women, particularly those who have had multiple pregnancies or are on hormone replacement therapy. A diet high in fat and cholesterol but low in fiber also plays a significant role in gallstone formation.

To mitigate these risks, individuals can adopt a balanced diet that emphasizes whole grains, fruits, vegetables, and lean proteins while reducing saturated fats and refined sugars. Regular physical activity is crucial, as it aids in maintaining a healthy weight and supports overall digestive health. Staying hydrated can also help in the prevention of gallstone formation.

CHAPTER 1:

Anatomy of the Gallbladder

Structure and Location of the Gallbladder

The gallbladder is a small, pear-shaped organ located beneath the liver in the upper right abdomen. It measures about 3 to 4 inches long and can hold approximately 30 to 50 milliliters of bile. Its anatomical position allows it to efficiently store bile produced by the liver until it is needed for digestion.

Understanding its structure is key to recognizing its role in digestion. The gallbladder has three main parts: the fundus (the rounded top), the body (the main portion), and the neck (which connects to the bile ducts). This structure enables the gallbladder to contract and release bile when needed.

Functions of the Gallbladder in the Digestive System

The primary function of the gallbladder is to store and concentrate bile, which is produced by the liver. Bile is a digestive fluid that helps break down fats, making it essential for the digestion of dietary lipids. When you eat a meal containing fat, the gallbladder contracts to release bile into the small intestine through the bile ducts.

In addition to storage, the gallbladder also concentrates bile by removing excess water. This process enhances the bile's effectiveness in digesting fats. By understanding this function, you can appreciate how gallbladder health is crucial for efficient digestion.

How Bile is Produced and Stored

Bile is produced continuously by the liver cells, known as hepatocytes. This process involves the synthesis of bile acids, cholesterol, bilirubin, and electrolytes. Once produced, bile flows through small ducts in the liver, converging into larger bile ducts that lead to the gallbladder for storage.

When you consume food, particularly fatty foods, hormones signal the gallbladder to release stored bile into the small intestine. This release is vital for emulsifying fats, making them easier for digestive enzymes to break down. Understanding this cycle helps you recognize how dietary habits can impact gallbladder function.

Role of the Gallbladder in Fat Digestion

The gallbladder plays a crucial role in fat digestion by releasing bile into the small intestine. Bile contains bile salts that emulsify fats, breaking them down into smaller droplets. This process increases the surface area of fats, allowing digestive enzymes, particularly lipases, to more effectively break down fat molecules into fatty acids and glycerol.

A well-functioning gallbladder ensures that enough bile is released when you eat fatty foods, which is essential for optimal digestion and nutrient absorption. Understanding this role highlights the importance of maintaining gallbladder health through a balanced diet.

Overview of Related Organs (Liver, Pancreas)

The liver and pancreas work in conjunction with the gallbladder to support digestion. The liver produces bile, which is stored in the gallbladder, while the pancreas secretes digestive enzymes and bicarbonate to neutralize stomach acid. Together, these organs create a harmonious system for digesting food.

In addition to digestion, the liver also processes nutrients absorbed from the intestine and detoxifies harmful substances. The pancreas regulates blood sugar levels by producing insulin and glucagon. Recognizing the interconnectedness of these organs can help you understand how gallbladder issues might affect overall health.

Importance of Gallbladder Health

Maintaining gallbladder health is vital for effective digestion and overall well-being. A healthy gallbladder helps ensure that bile is released when needed, allowing for proper fat digestion and absorption of fat-soluble vitamins (A, D, E, and K). Complications such as gallstones or inflammation can disrupt this process, leading to digestive issues.

To support gallbladder health, incorporate a balanced diet rich in fiber, healthy fats, and hydration. Regular exercise also promotes healthy digestion and bile flow. Understanding these aspects can empower you to take proactive steps for your gallbladder's well-being.

Common Symptoms of Gallbladder Issues

Common symptoms of gallbladder issues include abdominal pain, particularly in the upper right quadrant, bloating, nausea, and changes in bowel habits. Pain may occur after eating fatty meals, indicating that the gallbladder is struggling to release bile effectively. Recognizing these symptoms is crucial for early intervention.

If you experience persistent symptoms, it's essential to consult a healthcare provider. They may recommend further evaluation to determine the underlying cause, which could range from gallstones to gallbladder inflammation. Being aware of these symptoms enables you to seek help promptly.

Diagnostic Procedures for Gallbladder Disease

To diagnose gallbladder disease, healthcare providers may use several procedures, including ultrasound, CT scans, or MRIs. Ultrasound is the most common and non-invasive method, allowing doctors to visualize gallstones and assess gallbladder function. Blood tests can also help identify inflammation or infection.

If further evaluation is needed, providers may perform a HIDA scan to assess bile flow or an endoscopic retrograde cholangiopancreatography (ERCP) to visualize and potentially remove gallstones. Understanding these diagnostic tools helps demystify the process and prepares you for possible evaluations.

Understanding Bile and Its Components

Bile is a complex fluid composed mainly of bile salts, cholesterol, bilirubin, and phospholipids. Bile salts are derived from cholesterol and play a crucial role in emulsifying fats, while bilirubin is a waste product from the breakdown of red blood cells. Together, these components facilitate digestion and aid in the excretion of waste.

Recognizing the components of bile underscores its importance in digestion and liver health. A disruption in bile production or composition can lead to digestive issues and the formation of gallstones, making it vital to maintain a healthy liver and gallbladder.

Differences Between Healthy and Diseased Gallbladder

A healthy gallbladder efficiently stores and releases bile, allowing for optimal fat digestion. In contrast, a diseased gallbladder may have compromised function due to inflammation, gallstones, or other issues, leading to symptoms such as pain, bloating, and digestive disturbances.

Understanding these differences can help you recognize when to seek medical attention. If you notice changes in your digestion or experience discomfort, it's essential to discuss these with a healthcare provider for potential evaluations and treatment options.

Importance of Regular Check-Ups

Regular check-ups with a healthcare provider are crucial for maintaining gallbladder health. These appointments allow for early detection of potential issues, such as gallstones or inflammation, before they develop into more severe problems. Discussing any changes in symptoms or digestion during these visits can provide valuable insights.

Incorporating routine blood tests and imaging studies as recommended can help monitor gallbladder function. Understanding the importance of these check-ups empowers you to take charge of your health and proactively address any concerns.

Impact of Gallbladder Disease on Overall Health

Gallbladder disease can significantly impact overall health by disrupting the digestive process. Conditions such as gallstones or cholecystitis can lead to complications, including infections or pancreatitis, which may require more extensive medical intervention. Recognizing these potential risks can motivate individuals to prioritize their gallbladder health.

Maintaining a healthy diet and lifestyle can mitigate these risks and support gallbladder function. Understanding the interconnectedness of the gallbladder with other organs highlights the importance of addressing any issues promptly.

Lifestyle Factors Affecting Gallbladder Health

Several lifestyle factors can influence gallbladder health, including diet, physical activity, and hydration. A diet high in refined sugars and unhealthy fats can increase the risk of gallstone formation. Conversely, a balanced diet rich in fiber, whole grains, lean proteins, and healthy fats can support gallbladder function.

In addition to diet, regular physical activity promotes healthy digestion and helps maintain a healthy weight, reducing the risk of gallbladder disease. Staying hydrated is also essential, as it aids bile production and helps prevent gallstones. By understanding and modifying these lifestyle factors, individuals can take proactive steps toward better gallbladder health.

CHAPTER 2:

Causes of Gallbladder Disease

Detailed Overview of Gallstone Formation

Gallstones form when substances in the bile, primarily cholesterol and bilirubin, crystallize. This can occur when the liver produces too much cholesterol or bilirubin, or when the gallbladder does not empty efficiently. Understanding this process is crucial because it informs prevention strategies. In many cases, gallstones can remain asymptomatic for years before causing problems, often requiring diagnostic imaging for detection.

To better understand gallstone formation, consider the balance of components in bile. If the bile has too much cholesterol and not enough bile salts, the cholesterol may crystallize. Additionally, bilirubin can lead to pigment stones when produced in excess due to liver dysfunction. Maintaining a balanced diet can help regulate bile composition, thus reducing the risk of gallstones.

Risk Factors: Obesity, Diet, Age, and Gender

Obesity is a significant risk factor for gallstone formation as excess body weight can increase cholesterol levels in bile. Diets high in fat and low in fiber can further contribute to this risk. Age also plays a role, as gallstones are more common in individuals over 40, with hormonal changes in women during menopause increasing susceptibility.

Gender affects gallstone risk, with women more likely to develop them due to hormonal influences, particularly estrogen. Recognizing these risk factors allows for proactive lifestyle changes. For instance, adopting a balanced diet rich in fruits, vegetables, and whole grains can help mitigate these risks effectively.

Family History and Genetic Predisposition

A family history of gallstones can indicate a genetic predisposition to this condition. Certain genetic traits may affect cholesterol metabolism or gallbladder function, increasing the likelihood of stone formation. If gallstones are common in your family, it's essential to monitor your health closely and discuss concerns with a healthcare provider.

Understanding your family's health history empowers you to make informed lifestyle choices. Regular check-ups, maintaining a healthy weight, and a balanced diet can be particularly beneficial if gallstones run in your family. Genetic testing may also be an option for those with significant family histories of gallbladder disease.

How Pregnancy Affects Gallbladder Health

Pregnancy can impact gallbladder health due to hormonal changes that affect gallbladder motility. Increased levels of estrogen and progesterone can slow the gallbladder's ability to empty, raising the risk of gallstone formation. Moreover, physical changes during pregnancy can lead to increased pressure on the gallbladder, complicating its function.

To manage gallbladder health during pregnancy, it's crucial to maintain a well-balanced diet and stay hydrated. Eating smaller, more frequent meals may help prevent gallbladder complications. Pregnant individuals should consult their healthcare provider if they experience symptoms like abdominal pain or nausea, which could indicate gallbladder issues.

Other Medical Conditions Related to Gallbladder Disease

Certain medical conditions, such as liver disease, diabetes, and Crohn's disease, can increase the risk of gallbladder disease. For example, diabetes can lead to changes in cholesterol levels, potentially resulting in gallstones. Understanding these connections is vital for individuals with existing health conditions.

Managing these conditions through diet, regular check-ups, and medication adherence can help lower the risk of gallbladder problems. Collaborating with healthcare providers to monitor and manage these related conditions is essential in maintaining overall gallbladder health.

Medications That May Increase Gallstone Risk

Some medications, particularly hormone replacement therapy and cholesterol-lowering drugs, can increase the risk of gallstone formation. Medications that affect bile composition or gallbladder motility can lead to imbalances that promote stone development. It's important for patients to discuss their medication history with healthcare providers.

If you're taking medications that may increase gallstone risk, regular monitoring and consultation with your healthcare provider can help. Exploring alternative treatments or adjusting dosages may be options worth considering to minimize risks.

Understanding Cholesterol and Pigment Stones

Gallstones can be classified into two main types: cholesterol stones and pigment stones. Cholesterol stones, the most common type, form when there is excess cholesterol in the bile. Pigment stones, typically smaller and darker, result from excess bilirubin, often associated with conditions like liver cirrhosis or hemolytic anemia.

To manage the risk of both types of stones, dietary adjustments are crucial. Reducing saturated fats and increasing fiber intake can help lower cholesterol levels and reduce the likelihood of stone formation. Understanding the types of stones can guide dietary choices and preventive measures.

The Role of Fasting and Rapid Weight Loss

Fasting or undergoing rapid weight loss can significantly increase the risk of gallstone formation. When the body loses weight quickly, the liver secretes extra cholesterol into the bile, leading to stone formation. This is why slow, gradual weight loss is recommended for those needing to shed pounds.

To lose weight safely, aim for a balanced approach that includes regular physical activity and a nutritious diet. Gradual weight loss not only supports gallbladder health but also promotes long-term success in maintaining a healthy weight.

Importance of Dietary Habits

Diet plays a crucial role in gallbladder health, with certain foods promoting or hindering gallstone formation. Diets high in saturated fats and sugars increase the risk of cholesterol stones, while fiber-rich foods can help lower that risk. Incorporating fruits, vegetables, and whole grains is essential for maintaining a healthy bile composition.

To promote gallbladder health through diet, focus on balanced meals that include healthy fats, lean proteins, and complex carbohydrates. Being mindful of portion sizes and meal frequency can also aid in digestion and reduce the workload on the gallbladder.

Connection Between Gallbladder Disease and Diabetes

There is a notable connection between gallbladder disease and diabetes. Individuals with diabetes often have altered cholesterol metabolism, increasing the likelihood of gallstones. Additionally, insulin resistance may impact gallbladder function, further complicating the health of the gallbladder.

Managing blood sugar levels through a balanced diet and regular exercise can help mitigate this risk. Regular check-ups and open communication with healthcare providers about gallbladder health are vital for those with diabetes.

Lifestyle Changes to Reduce Risk

Making lifestyle changes can significantly reduce the risk of gallbladder disease. Regular physical activity, maintaining a healthy weight, and adopting a balanced diet are essential steps. Limiting high-fat, high-sugar foods can help maintain optimal bile composition, reducing the risk of stone formation.

Incorporating simple changes, such as walking daily or preparing healthier meals at home, can create significant improvements over time. These lifestyle adjustments not only promote gallbladder health but also contribute to overall well-being.

Recognizing Early Signs of Gallbladder Problems

Early recognition of gallbladder problems can lead to timely intervention. Common symptoms include pain in the upper right abdomen, especially after fatty meals, nausea, and bloating. Keeping track of these symptoms can help individuals seek medical advice promptly.

If you notice any persistent symptoms or changes in your digestive health, it's essential to consult a healthcare provider. Early detection can facilitate better management and potentially avoid complications associated with gallbladder disease.

Seeking Medical Advice When Symptoms Occur

When experiencing symptoms of gallbladder disease, seeking medical advice is crucial. A healthcare provider can evaluate symptoms through physical examinations, imaging tests, and lab work. Early diagnosis can significantly affect the management of gallbladder conditions.

If diagnosed with gallbladder disease or gallstones, working closely with a healthcare provider to develop a treatment plan tailored to your needs is essential. This may include lifestyle changes, dietary adjustments, or exploring medical and surgical options to address the condition effectively.

CHAPTER 3:

Symptoms of Gallbladder Disease

Common Symptoms: Pain, Nausea, and Vomiting

Gallbladder disease often presents with a few key symptoms, primarily pain in the upper right abdomen, nausea, and vomiting. The pain can range from mild discomfort to severe cramping, especially after consuming fatty foods. Recognizing these symptoms early is crucial, as they can indicate the presence of gallstones or inflammation in the gallbladder. Keeping a symptom diary can help you identify patterns related to your diet and activity levels.

In addition to pain, nausea and vomiting may accompany gallbladder issues, particularly during a gallbladder attack. These symptoms can lead to significant distress and may affect your appetite and ability to eat. If you frequently experience these symptoms, consider consulting a healthcare provider for evaluation and possible dietary adjustments to manage your symptoms better.

Location of Pain Associated with Gallbladder Issues

Gallbladder pain typically occurs in the upper right abdomen, just below the rib cage, and can radiate to the back or right shoulder. This pain is often sharp or cramping, especially after meals, particularly those high in fat. Understanding the location of this pain can help you and your healthcare provider determine if gallbladder disease is the cause, facilitating timely diagnosis and treatment.

When experiencing gallbladder-related pain, it may be beneficial to note the timing and duration of your discomfort. Documenting when the pain occurs—such as after specific meals—can provide valuable information to your doctor. This can lead to more effective treatment options and dietary changes that help reduce the occurrence of pain.

Understanding Acute vs. Chronic Symptoms

Acute symptoms of gallbladder disease manifest suddenly and can include severe abdominal pain, nausea, and vomiting. These symptoms often indicate a gallbladder attack or acute cholecystitis, which may require immediate medical attention. If you experience sudden and intense pain, especially if it lasts more than a few hours, it's essential to seek medical help right away.

Chronic symptoms, on the other hand, develop gradually and can include intermittent pain, bloating, and indigestion. These symptoms may not always indicate a gallbladder attack but can be equally troublesome. Monitoring your symptoms over time can help you understand whether they are acute or chronic, guiding your approach to management and treatment.

When to Seek Medical Attention

It is crucial to know when to seek medical attention for gallbladder disease. You should contact a healthcare provider if you experience severe abdominal pain that lasts more than a few hours, fever, jaundice (yellowing of the skin or eyes), or persistent nausea and vomiting. These signs may indicate a more serious condition that requires prompt intervention, such as a blocked bile duct or infection.

Additionally, if your symptoms interfere with daily activities or worsen over time, it's time to consult a healthcare professional. Early diagnosis and treatment can prevent complications and lead to better outcomes. Don't hesitate to reach out to your doctor if you are unsure about your symptoms; timely evaluation can make a significant difference.

Differentiating Between Gallbladder Pain and Other Abdominal Pain

Differentiating gallbladder pain from other types of abdominal pain can be challenging. Gallbladder pain is typically located in the upper right quadrant of the abdomen and may radiate to the back or shoulder. It often occurs after eating, particularly after fatty meals, which can help distinguish it from other conditions like acid reflux or gastric ulcers.

To help identify gallbladder pain, pay attention to accompanying symptoms such as nausea, vomiting, or changes in bowel habits. Keeping a detailed record of your symptoms and their timing can aid in this differentiation and provide valuable information to your healthcare provider during your evaluation.

Potential Complications if Left Untreated

Untreated gallbladder disease can lead to serious complications, including cholecystitis (inflammation of the gallbladder), pancreatitis, and biliary obstruction. Cholecystitis occurs when gallstones block the ducts, causing severe pain and infection, while pancreatitis can arise if a gallstone obstructs the pancreatic duct. Both conditions require immediate medical attention.

In addition to these complications, untreated gallbladder disease can lead to the formation of more gallstones and increased pain episodes. Regular check-ups and monitoring of symptoms can help prevent these complications. Discussing potential risks with your healthcare provider allows you to make informed decisions about your treatment plan and lifestyle adjustments.

Importance of Symptom Tracking

Tracking your symptoms is an essential part of managing gallbladder disease. Keeping a symptom diary helps identify patterns and triggers associated with your pain and discomfort. Note when symptoms occur, their duration, and any dietary or lifestyle factors that may influence them. This information can assist your healthcare provider in diagnosing and tailoring treatment strategies.

By systematically recording your symptoms, you can also evaluate the effectiveness of any dietary adjustments or treatments. This proactive approach can lead to more personalized care and improved quality of life. Regular updates to your healthcare provider about your symptom tracking can enhance their understanding of your condition and guide future recommendations.

The Role of Imaging Tests in Symptom Assessment

Imaging tests, such as ultrasound, CT scans, or MRI, are crucial in assessing gallbladder disease. These tests help visualize the gallbladder, identify the presence of gallstones, and determine any inflammation or blockage. Ultrasound is typically the first-line imaging test due to its non-invasive nature and effectiveness in detecting gallstones.

Understanding the role of imaging can help alleviate anxiety associated with the diagnosis process. These tests are usually quick, and results are typically available shortly after. Engaging in discussions with your healthcare provider about what to expect during these tests can enhance your comfort and preparedness for the assessment.

Overview of Gallbladder Attacks

A gallbladder attack, often due to gallstones blocking the bile ducts, results in severe abdominal pain, typically in the upper right quadrant. This attack can occur suddenly and may be accompanied by nausea, vomiting, and sweating. Recognizing the onset of a gallbladder attack is crucial for managing the pain and seeking timely medical assistance.

To manage a gallbladder attack, it's advisable to rest in a comfortable position and apply a warm compress to the abdomen to alleviate discomfort. Over-the-counter pain relief may also be beneficial, but consult with your healthcare provider for recommendations tailored to your specific situation. If symptoms persist or worsen, seek medical attention immediately to prevent complications.

Symptoms of Gallstone Complications (e.g., Pancreatitis)

Gallstones can lead to serious complications, such as pancreatitis, characterized by severe abdominal pain, nausea, vomiting, and fever. Pancreatitis occurs when gallstones obstruct the pancreatic duct, leading to inflammation and potential damage to the pancreas. Recognizing the symptoms of complications early is essential to ensure prompt treatment and prevent further health issues.

If you experience symptoms suggestive of pancreatitis, such as intense upper abdominal pain that may radiate to the back, seek medical attention immediately. Early intervention can help manage the condition and reduce the risk of severe complications, including organ failure. Keeping your healthcare provider informed about any sudden changes in your symptoms is crucial for effective management.

Understanding Silent Gallstones

Silent gallstones are gallstones that do not cause noticeable symptoms. Many people may have these stones without knowing, as they do not experience any pain or discomfort. However, silent gallstones can still lead to complications if they block bile ducts or become inflamed. Regular check-ups with your healthcare provider can help monitor for any changes in your condition.

If diagnosed with silent gallstones, your healthcare provider may recommend a watchful waiting approach, especially if you're not experiencing symptoms. However, it's essential to stay vigilant and report any new or unusual symptoms promptly. Discussing the best course of action with your healthcare provider will help ensure your health remains a priority.

The Impact of Symptoms on Daily Life

Gallbladder disease can significantly impact daily life, causing disruptions in activities and overall well-being. Symptoms such as pain, nausea, and digestive issues may prevent individuals from participating in social events or enjoying meals, leading to feelings of isolation or frustration. Understanding this impact is vital for developing effective coping strategies.

To manage the daily effects of gallbladder disease, consider making dietary adjustments to avoid triggers and enhance digestive health. Regularly practicing relaxation techniques, such as deep breathing or gentle exercise, can also alleviate stress related to managing symptoms. Seeking support from healthcare professionals, friends, or support groups can further aid in navigating the challenges of living with gallbladder disease.

Coping Strategies for Managing Symptoms

Managing symptoms of gallbladder disease involves various coping strategies. Dietary changes, such as reducing fat intake and increasing fiber, can help alleviate symptoms. Eating smaller, more frequent meals rather than large ones can also ease digestive strain. Keeping a food diary to identify specific triggers can guide your dietary choices effectively.

In addition to dietary adjustments, lifestyle modifications play a crucial role in symptom management. Regular physical activity can help maintain a healthy weight and improve digestion. Stress management techniques, such as mindfulness or yoga, can reduce overall discomfort and enhance your quality of life. Engaging in regular check-ups with your healthcare provider will also help monitor your condition and adjust your management plan as necessary.

CHAPTER 4:

Diagnosis of Gallbladder Disease

Overview of Diagnostic Tests for Gallbladder Disease

Diagnosing gallbladder disease typically involves a combination of imaging and laboratory tests that help determine the presence of gallstones, inflammation, or other abnormalities. Your healthcare provider will start by reviewing your symptoms, which may include abdominal pain, nausea, and digestive issues. Based on your symptoms and medical history, they will recommend specific tests to confirm the diagnosis.

Common diagnostic tests include ultrasound, blood tests, and various imaging techniques. Each of these tests plays a crucial role in understanding the function of your gallbladder and the surrounding organs. It's essential to follow your healthcare provider's recommendations for these tests to ensure accurate diagnosis and timely treatment.

Ultrasound as the Primary Diagnostic Tool

Ultrasound is often the first test performed when gallbladder disease is suspected. It uses sound waves to create images of the gallbladder and surrounding structures, allowing healthcare providers to detect gallstones, inflammation, or any other abnormalities. The procedure is non-invasive, painless, and usually takes about 30 minutes.

During the ultrasound, you may be asked to lie on your back while a technician applies a gel to your abdomen and moves a small handheld device (transducer) over the area. If gallstones are present, they will appear as bright white spots on the images. Ultrasound is particularly effective because it does not expose you to radiation, making it safe for most patients.

Other Imaging Tests: CT Scans, MRIs, and HIDA Scans

If ultrasound results are inconclusive, your doctor may recommend additional imaging tests like CT scans, MRIs, or HIDA scans. A CT scan uses X-rays to produce detailed cross-sectional images of your abdomen, allowing for a more thorough evaluation of the gallbladder and nearby organs. MRI, on the other hand, uses magnetic fields and radio waves to create images, providing detailed information about soft tissues.

A HIDA scan involves injecting a small amount of radioactive dye into your bloodstream, which then travels to the liver and gallbladder. This test helps assess how well your gallbladder is functioning. Each imaging test has its specific advantages, and your healthcare provider will choose the best option based on your individual situation.

Blood Tests for Assessing Liver and Gallbladder Function

Blood tests are essential for evaluating liver and gallbladder function, helping to identify underlying issues related to gallbladder disease. Common tests include liver function tests (LFTs), which measure the levels of various enzymes, proteins, and substances produced by the liver. Elevated levels may indicate inflammation or obstruction.

In addition to LFTs, your doctor may order a complete blood count (CBC) to check for signs of infection or anemia. These tests provide valuable information that complements imaging studies, helping your healthcare provider develop a comprehensive understanding of your health status and guide appropriate treatment.

Importance of a Thorough Medical History

A thorough medical history is critical for diagnosing gallbladder disease. When you meet with your healthcare provider, be prepared to discuss your symptoms, medical background, and any family history of gallbladder issues. This information helps your doctor identify risk factors and tailor diagnostic approaches accordingly.

Be honest about any medications you take, dietary habits, and lifestyle factors that could influence gallbladder health. This comprehensive approach aids in pinpointing potential causes of your symptoms and ensures that you receive the most accurate diagnosis and effective treatment plan.

Physical Examination Findings

During a physical examination, your healthcare provider will assess your abdomen for tenderness or pain, particularly in the upper right quadrant where the gallbladder is located. They may also check for signs of jaundice (yellowing of the skin and eyes) or other indicators of liver dysfunction.

Your doctor will evaluate your overall health by asking about your symptoms and any previous medical conditions. This examination, combined with your medical history and diagnostic tests, provides a complete picture of your gallbladder health, guiding further evaluations or treatment options.

Role of Endoscopic Procedures

Endoscopic procedures, such as endoscopic retrograde cholangiopancreatography (ERCP), are vital for diagnosing and treating gallbladder disease, particularly when there is suspicion of bile duct obstruction. During ERCP, a thin tube with a camera is inserted through the mouth and into the duodenum to visualize the bile ducts.

If gallstones are detected in the bile ducts during this procedure, the doctor can often remove them at the same time. This minimally invasive approach can help alleviate symptoms and prevent complications without the need for more invasive surgery.

Interpreting Test Results

Interpreting test results is a crucial step in diagnosing gallbladder disease. Your healthcare provider will analyze the findings from imaging studies, blood tests, and any endoscopic procedures to determine the presence and extent of any gallbladder issues. It's essential to discuss the significance of these results with your provider, as they will guide your treatment options.

Understanding your test results can help you make informed decisions about your health. If there are any abnormalities, your doctor will explain what they mean and discuss the next steps in your management plan, whether that involves dietary changes, medications, or surgical interventions.

When Further Evaluation is Needed

In some cases, further evaluation may be necessary if initial tests do not provide a clear diagnosis. This could involve repeat imaging tests, additional blood work, or specialized procedures to gain more insights into your condition. Your healthcare provider will discuss the reasons for further evaluation and outline the necessary steps.

Recognizing when to seek further evaluation is important for timely diagnosis and treatment. If symptoms persist or worsen, or if new symptoms develop, it's essential to communicate these changes to your healthcare provider promptly.

The Significance of Early Diagnosis

Early diagnosis of gallbladder disease is crucial for preventing complications, such as infection or gallbladder rupture. Detecting gallstones or inflammation early on allows for timely interventions that can alleviate symptoms and prevent more severe issues down the line. Being proactive about your health can significantly improve outcomes.

To facilitate early diagnosis, pay attention to any warning signs and maintain regular check-ups with your healthcare provider. If you experience persistent abdominal pain, nausea, or other concerning symptoms, seek medical advice promptly to ensure appropriate evaluation and management.

Discussing Diagnosis with Your Healthcare Provider

Having open discussions with your healthcare provider about your diagnosis is essential. Ask questions about your condition, the implications of your test results, and the recommended treatment options. A clear understanding of your diagnosis will help you feel more empowered in managing your health.

Being informed allows you to actively participate in your care plan. Don't hesitate to voice any concerns or preferences regarding treatment options, as collaborative decision-making can lead to better outcomes and a more personalized approach to your healthcare.

Understanding the Implications of Test Findings

Understanding the implications of test findings is key to managing gallbladder disease effectively. Each result provides insights into your gallbladder's health and informs potential treatment strategies. For instance, the presence of gallstones may necessitate lifestyle changes, medication, or surgical intervention, depending on the severity of your symptoms.

Discuss the meaning of your test results with your healthcare provider to gain a clear perspective on your condition.

Preparing for Diagnostic Tests

Preparing for diagnostic tests involves following specific instructions provided by your healthcare provider to ensure accurate results. For example, some tests may require fasting for several hours before the procedure, while others may need you to avoid certain medications. Adhering to these guidelines is crucial for obtaining reliable data.

Additionally, it may be helpful to write down any questions or concerns you have before your appointment. Being well-prepared not only helps you understand the process better but also ensures that you make the most of your healthcare provider's expertise during the diagnostic evaluation.

CHAPTER 5:

Treatment Options for Gallbladder Disease

Overview of Treatment Approaches for Gallbladder Disease

Treatment for gallbladder disease typically begins with non-invasive approaches, especially for mild cases, such as dietary changes and medications to manage symptoms. For more severe cases, medical professionals may recommend non-surgical treatments like lithotripsy or surgical options, such as removing the gallbladder entirely. Understanding these various approaches allows individuals to make informed decisions on what might work best for their unique situation, with guidance from healthcare providers.

In general, the goal of gallbladder disease treatment is to manage symptoms, prevent further complications, and maintain overall health. From medications to lifestyle adjustments, patients should consult with a medical professional to explore these options fully. This comprehensive approach allows patients to find the most effective treatments for their specific needs and optimize their overall well-being.

Dietary Modifications as a First-Line Treatment

Dietary changes can be a powerful first-line treatment for gallbladder disease. Reducing intake of high-fat and fried foods can lessen strain on the gallbladder, helping to prevent painful attacks and improve digestion. Including fiber-rich foods, like fruits, vegetables, and whole grains, also supports digestive health and can reduce the likelihood of gallstone formation.

For individuals with gallbladder issues, small, frequent meals may help in managing symptoms and preventing bile build-up. By making conscious, balanced food choices, patients can effectively manage and often reduce gallbladder disease symptoms without requiring more invasive interventions.

Non-Surgical vs. Surgical Interventions

Non-surgical options for gallbladder disease typically include medication, lifestyle modifications, and sometimes shock wave therapy to break down gallstones. These approaches can be effective for mild cases, especially when gallstones are small and cause fewer symptoms. Non-surgical interventions aim to manage discomfort while preserving the gallbladder when possible.

On the other hand, surgical options, such as a cholecystectomy, are often recommended when non-surgical treatments are ineffective or when gallstones lead to more severe complications. This procedure removes the gallbladder, which can permanently resolve symptoms and prevent future gallstone formation. Deciding between these options depends on the individual's specific condition and the severity of their symptoms.

Understanding the Role of Medications

Medications for gallbladder disease typically aim to dissolve gallstones, reduce inflammation, or relieve pain associated with gallstone attacks. Ursodeoxycholic acid, for example, can help dissolve certain types of gallstones and is commonly prescribed for patients seeking non-surgical treatment options. Pain medications are also frequently recommended to manage discomfort during gallbladder attacks.

While medications can be effective for some, they may not be a long-term solution, particularly if gallstones continue to form or cause recurrent issues. Patients should work closely with their healthcare providers to understand the benefits and limitations of medication and to determine if additional treatments are needed.

Introduction to Laparoscopic Cholecystectomy

Laparoscopic cholecystectomy is a minimally invasive surgical procedure to remove the gallbladder. During this procedure, small incisions are made in the abdomen through which a tiny camera and surgical tools are inserted. The surgeon then removes the gallbladder with minimal impact on surrounding tissues. Laparoscopic cholecystectomy generally has a shorter recovery time compared to open surgery, allowing most patients to resume normal activities within a week.

This surgery is commonly recommended for those with severe or recurring gallstone attacks, as it offers a permanent solution by removing the gallbladder. Patients should discuss with their surgeons what to expect during and after the procedure to ensure a smooth recovery and optimal outcome.

Post-Operative Care and Recovery

Following a laparoscopic cholecystectomy, patients are typically encouraged to rest and avoid strenuous activities for a week. During recovery, it's important to monitor for signs of infection at the incision sites, such as redness or swelling, and to follow any dietary guidelines provided by the healthcare team. A low-fat diet is often recommended initially to help the digestive system adjust.

Most people can resume normal activities relatively quickly, but it's essential to follow the specific recovery plan laid out by the surgeon. Attending follow-up appointments ensures that recovery is progressing well and that there are no post-operative complications.

Potential Complications of Surgery

While laparoscopic cholecystectomy is generally safe, potential complications include infections, bile duct injuries, and bleeding. Symptoms such as fever, severe abdominal pain, or persistent nausea following surgery may indicate complications that require immediate medical attention. Patients should be aware of these risks and know when to seek help if symptoms arise post-surgery.

Although complications are rare, discussing them with a healthcare provider can help patients make an informed decision. Surgeons usually outline preventive steps and provide guidance on minimizing risks, ensuring patients feel prepared and supported throughout the surgical process.

Alternative Treatments and Their Effectiveness

Alternative treatments, such as herbal remedies, acupuncture, and bile salt supplements, are sometimes explored by patients seeking non-medical options for managing gallbladder disease. These methods may offer temporary symptom relief, particularly for mild cases, but they are not substitutes for traditional treatments like medication or surgery.

It's essential to approach alternative treatments with caution and consult a healthcare provider before trying them. While some patients may find complementary therapies helpful, their effectiveness varies, and they may not address the root cause of gallbladder disease or prevent future complications.

Importance of Personalized Treatment Plans

Each individual's experience with gallbladder disease is unique, making personalized treatment plans crucial for effective management. Factors like age, overall health, and the severity of symptoms play a role in determining the best course of action. Working closely with a healthcare provider ensures that the treatment approach aligns with personal health goals and addresses specific needs.

Personalized plans also offer flexibility, allowing adjustments based on how the patient responds to treatment. This tailored approach enhances the likelihood of successful symptom management and improved quality of life.

Role of Support Groups and Resources

Support groups can be invaluable for individuals managing gallbladder disease, offering emotional support, shared experiences, and practical advice. Connecting with others who understand the challenges of gallbladder disease can provide a sense of comfort and reduce feelings of isolation. Online forums, in-person meetings, and patient advocacy organizations often facilitate these connections.

In addition to support groups, resources like dietary guides, educational materials, and medical websites can help patients stay informed about managing their condition. These tools enable individuals to take an active role in their health and feel empowered throughout their treatment journey.

Monitoring and Follow-Up Care After Treatment

Regular follow-up care is essential for monitoring any lingering symptoms or potential complications after gallbladder treatment. During follow-up visits, healthcare providers may assess digestive function, evaluate recovery progress, and address any ongoing concerns the patient may have. These appointments also offer an opportunity to adjust dietary and lifestyle recommendations based on the patient's recovery experience.

Maintaining open communication with healthcare providers ensures that patients receive ongoing support and guidance. Consistent follow-up helps to catch any issues early, facilitating timely interventions if needed for optimal long-term health.

Strategies for Managing Chronic Gallbladder Disease

For individuals with chronic gallbladder disease, long-term management strategies focus on lifestyle changes and regular monitoring to prevent flare-ups. This may include a balanced, low-fat diet, stress management techniques, and staying hydrated. Regular physical activity can also aid digestion and support overall gallbladder health.

Adopting these strategies helps individuals maintain a stable routine that minimizes symptoms and enhances their quality of life. Working with healthcare providers to develop a sustainable plan can make managing chronic gallbladder disease more manageable and less disruptive.

Integrating Treatment into Daily Life

Integrating gallbladder disease management into daily routines involves a combination of dietary adjustments, regular medication (if prescribed), and mindful eating habits. Preparing low-fat meals ahead of time and having healthy snacks on hand can help avoid situations that may trigger gallbladder attacks. Additionally, paying attention to portion sizes and eating smaller meals can ease the digestive load on the body.

Creating a lifestyle that supports gallbladder health helps individuals navigate their day-to-day activities with minimal interruption from symptoms. Staying consistent with these practices empowers patients to manage their condition more effectively while maintaining a fulfilling, active life.

CHAPTER 6:

Dietary Adjustments for Gallbladder Health

Importance of a Gallbladder-Friendly Diet

A gallbladder-friendly diet is crucial for maintaining optimal digestive health and preventing complications associated with gallbladder disease, particularly gallstones. By focusing on nutrient-rich foods, you can support your body's digestion and minimize symptoms like bloating and discomfort. A well-balanced diet can help reduce the risk of gallstones and support overall gallbladder function, which is essential for processing fats and nutrients effectively.

When designing a gallbladder-friendly diet, it's vital to prioritize whole, unprocessed foods while minimizing high-fat and sugary options. This approach not only helps manage symptoms but can also enhance your overall well-being, making it easier for your body to function correctly. Small dietary changes can lead to significant improvements in your gallbladder health and overall quality of life.

Foods to Include: Fruits, Vegetables, and Whole Grains

Incorporating a variety of fruits, vegetables, and whole grains into your diet is essential for gallbladder health. These foods are rich in vitamins, minerals, and antioxidants, which support digestion and promote overall wellness. Aim to fill half your plate with colorful fruits and vegetables at each meal, ensuring a broad spectrum of nutrients. Whole grains, such as brown rice, quinoa, and whole wheat bread, provide essential fiber, which can help keep your digestive system functioning smoothly.

When selecting fruits and vegetables, focus on options that are high in fiber and low in fat. Apples, pears, berries, leafy greens, and broccoli are excellent choices. By including these foods in your meals and snacks, you can create a satisfying and nutritious diet that supports gallbladder health while also helping to manage weight.

Foods to Avoid: Saturated Fats and Refined Sugars

To protect your gallbladder, it's essential to avoid foods high in saturated fats and refined sugars, which can contribute to gallstone formation and digestive discomfort. Saturated fats are often found in fatty meats, full-fat dairy products, and processed foods. Instead, opt for lean protein sources, such as chicken, turkey, and fish, which provide essential nutrients without putting unnecessary stress on your gallbladder.

Refined sugars, commonly found in sugary drinks, desserts, and many processed snacks, can lead to weight gain and increased cholesterol levels, further heightening the risk of gallstones. Focus on natural sweeteners like honey or maple syrup in moderation and choose whole, unprocessed foods whenever possible to maintain balanced blood sugar levels and promote gallbladder health.

Understanding the Role of Fiber in Digestion

Fiber plays a vital role in digestion by promoting regular bowel movements and preventing constipation, which is especially important for gallbladder health. Soluble fiber, found in foods like oats, beans, and fruits, helps to bind cholesterol and prevent its absorption into the bloodstream, reducing the risk of gallstone formation. Insoluble fiber, found in whole grains and vegetables, adds bulk to the stool, making it easier to pass.

To incorporate more fiber into your diet, gradually increase your intake of high-fiber foods while drinking plenty of water to avoid digestive discomfort. Aim for at least 25-30 grams of fiber daily, and try to include a variety of sources to reap the benefits of both soluble and insoluble fiber. This approach will support your digestive system and help maintain gallbladder health.

Meal Planning Tips for Gallbladder Health

Effective meal planning is key to maintaining a gallbladder-friendly diet. Start by creating a weekly meal schedule that includes a balance of fruits, vegetables, whole grains, and lean proteins. Planning your meals in advance allows you to choose nutritious options, avoiding impulse buys and unhealthy choices. Consider batch cooking or prepping meals to save time and ensure that healthy options are readily available throughout the week.

When planning meals, be mindful of portion sizes to avoid overeating, which can strain the gallbladder. Use smaller plates to help control serving sizes, and listen to your body's hunger cues. This approach will not only help you maintain a healthy diet but also support your gallbladder function and overall digestive health.

Importance of Hydration

Staying hydrated is essential for overall health, including gallbladder function. Proper hydration helps to maintain bile consistency, which is crucial for fat digestion and the prevention of gallstone formation. Aim to drink at least 8 cups (64 ounces) of water per day, adjusting for activity level and climate. Herbal teas and infused water can also be great alternatives to keep your fluid intake interesting and enjoyable.

To monitor your hydration levels, pay attention to the color of your urine; it should be light yellow. If it's dark or concentrated, increase your fluid intake. Staying adequately hydrated will not only support your gallbladder health but also improve your digestion and overall well-being.

Incorporating Healthy Fats into Your Diet

Incorporating healthy fats into your diet is crucial for gallbladder health. Healthy fats, such as those found in avocados, nuts, seeds, and fatty fish, can help regulate cholesterol levels and promote bile production, essential for digesting fats. Aim to include sources of healthy fats in moderation, as they provide essential fatty acids that support cellular function and overall health.

To include healthy fats in your meals, try adding slices of avocado to salads, snacking on a handful of nuts, or cooking with olive oil instead of butter. This approach not only enhances the flavor of your meals but also provides the necessary nutrients your body needs without putting unnecessary strain on your gallbladder.

Sample Meal Ideas for Gallbladder Health

Creating delicious and nutritious meals for gallbladder health can be straightforward. For breakfast, consider oatmeal topped with fresh berries and a sprinkle of nuts for added fiber and healthy fats. A lunch option might be a quinoa salad with mixed greens, chickpeas, cucumbers, and a light vinaigrette. Dinner can include grilled salmon with steamed broccoli and brown rice for a balanced and satisfying meal.

Snacks are also essential in a gallbladder-friendly diet; try hummus with carrot sticks, Greek yogurt with fruit, or apple slices with almond butter. By mixing and matching these meal ideas, you can ensure a diverse and enjoyable diet that supports your gallbladder health while keeping your taste buds satisfied.

The Role of Portion Control

Portion control is essential in managing gallbladder disease, as overeating can trigger symptoms and put extra strain on the digestive system. To practice portion control, consider using smaller plates and bowls to create the illusion of a fuller plate. Additionally, aim to fill half your plate with vegetables, one quarter with lean protein, and one quarter with whole grains for a balanced meal.

Listening to your body's hunger and fullness signals is equally important. Eat slowly and take time to savor each bite, allowing your brain to register when you're satisfied. This mindful approach will help prevent overeating and ensure your gallbladder remains healthy.

How to Read Food Labels Effectively

Learning to read food labels effectively is a valuable skill for maintaining a gallbladder-friendly diet. Start by checking the serving size, as it determines the nutritional information provided. Look for products that are low in saturated fats and sugars while being high in fiber, protein, and healthy fats. Familiarize yourself with terms like "trans fat" and "cholesterol" to make informed choices.

In addition to the nutrition facts, examine the ingredient list. The fewer ingredients, the better, as whole foods tend to be more nutritious than processed ones. Prioritize products with recognizable ingredients and avoid those with artificial additives or high levels of refined sugars, helping you make better food choices that support gallbladder health.

The Impact of Caffeine and Alcohol on Gallbladder Health

Caffeine and alcohol can significantly impact gallbladder health, so it's important to consume them in moderation or avoid them altogether. Caffeine, found in coffee and certain teas, may stimulate the gallbladder, leading to contractions that can cause discomfort for some individuals. If you notice symptoms after consuming caffeinated beverages, consider switching to herbal teas or decaffeinated options.

Alcohol can also contribute to gallbladder problems, as excessive consumption can lead to inflammation and increase the risk of gallstones. To promote gallbladder health, limit alcohol intake to moderate levels, which is defined as up to one drink per day for women and two for men. By being mindful of your consumption, you can better manage your gallbladder health.

Strategies for Dining Out While Managing Gallbladder Disease

Dining out can be challenging for individuals managing gallbladder disease, but with some strategies, it can still be enjoyable. Before going out, review the restaurant's menu online and look for gallbladder-friendly options such as grilled or baked dishes, salads, and whole grains. Don't hesitate to ask the server about modifications to make meals healthier, such as dressing on the side or substituting fried items for steamed vegetables.

While at the restaurant, practice portion control by sharing dishes or ordering smaller portions. Focus on enjoying the dining experience rather than just the food; this mindful approach can help you avoid overeating. By planning ahead and making informed choices, you can enjoy dining out without compromising your gallbladder health.

Importance of Consulting with a Dietitian

Consulting with a registered dietitian is invaluable for individuals managing gallbladder disease. A dietitian can help tailor a personalized meal plan that considers your specific dietary needs, preferences, and health goals. They can also provide guidance on making dietary adjustments and educate you about which foods to include or avoid for optimal gallbladder health.

Working with a dietitian can also offer ongoing support, motivation, and accountability, making it easier to adhere to your dietary plan. They can help you navigate challenges, answer questions, and provide strategies for maintaining a balanced and nutritious diet, ultimately leading to better health outcomes.

CHAPTER 7:

Lifestyle Changes for Gallbladder Disease

The Role of Exercise in Gallbladder Health

Exercise plays a key role in keeping the gallbladder functioning properly by stimulating the digestive system and helping to prevent the buildup of cholesterol, which can lead to gallstones. Regular physical activities such as walking, cycling, and swimming encourage bile flow and assist in fat breakdown, reducing strain on the gallbladder. Aim for at least 30 minutes of moderate exercise most days of the week to keep your gallbladder in good shape.

Additionally, engaging in strength training a couple of times a week can support metabolism and help maintain a healthy weight, which further reduces the risk of gallbladder disease. Stretching exercises, yoga, and Pilates can be added to your routine to improve flexibility, support organ function, and promote overall well-being. Making exercise a consistent part of your routine is beneficial not only for gallbladder health but also for general digestive health and well-being.

Importance of Maintaining a Healthy Weight

Maintaining a healthy weight is crucial for gallbladder health, as excess body fat can increase cholesterol levels in bile, leading to gallstone formation. A balanced diet rich in fiber, lean protein, and healthy fats helps manage weight effectively and supports the digestive system. Focus on portion control, minimize sugary and fatty foods, and include plenty of fruits and vegetables to support a healthy weight and promote gallbladder function.

To maintain a steady weight, aim for gradual weight loss if needed, as rapid weight loss can actually increase the risk of gallstones. Strive for a balanced approach to dieting, including regular physical activity and nutritious meals, to avoid stressing the gallbladder and keep it functioning optimally. Consistent, small changes to your lifestyle can have long-lasting benefits for both weight management and gallbladder health.

Stress Management Techniques and Their Impact on Digestion

Stress can interfere with digestion and bile production, making stress management essential for gallbladder health. Practices such as deep breathing, meditation, and mindfulness can help calm the nervous system, reducing the risk of stress-induced digestive issues. Allocate a few minutes each day for relaxation exercises to help improve digestion and support gallbladder function.

Creating a stress-relief routine that includes activities like journaling, gentle exercises, or even talking to a friend can further improve digestion and overall health. Managing stress through these methods promotes a healthy digestive system and can reduce symptoms associated with gallbladder problems, making it easier for your body to process food without added strain on the gallbladder.

Strategies for Improving Sleep Quality

Good sleep is essential for gallbladder health, as poor sleep can disrupt digestion and increase stress hormones, affecting bile production and increasing the risk of gallstones. Establish a consistent sleep routine by going to bed and waking up at the same time each day. Limit caffeine, alcohol, and heavy meals in the evening to promote better sleep quality and overall digestive health.

Creating a restful sleep environment can also make a big difference. Keep your bedroom dark, cool, and quiet, and avoid screens for at least an hour before bed. Developing healthy sleep habits will not only support your gallbladder but will also improve your overall well-being by enhancing your body's ability to repair and restore overnight.

Understanding the Link Between Smoking and Gallbladder Disease

Smoking can significantly impact gallbladder health by increasing cholesterol levels in the bile and promoting inflammation, both of which raise the risk of gallstones. Quitting smoking reduces these risks and can help restore balance to your digestive system. Support for quitting smoking, such as counseling, nicotine replacement therapy, or support groups, can be highly effective in helping you make the change.

Additionally, avoiding exposure to secondhand smoke can further protect the gallbladder and overall health. By eliminating smoking from your lifestyle, you can enhance not only your gallbladder function but also your overall cardiovascular and respiratory health, reducing the likelihood of complications related to gallbladder disease.

Importance of Regular Health Check-Ups

Regular health check-ups are vital for early detection of gallbladder issues, such as gallstones or inflammation, which can be managed more effectively when caught early. During these check-ups, your healthcare provider may perform an ultrasound or blood tests to monitor your gallbladder function and ensure there are no issues with bile production or flow.

These check-ups also provide an opportunity to discuss any digestive symptoms, dietary changes, or lifestyle habits that may impact gallbladder health. Staying proactive with annual check-ups allows you to address potential concerns early and implement preventive measures to maintain a healthy gallbladder and overall digestive system.

Developing a Support Network

Having a support network can be incredibly beneficial when managing gallbladder health, as friends and family can provide encouragement and accountability. Sharing your health goals with close ones and engaging in healthy activities together can make lifestyle changes easier and more enjoyable. Whether it's cooking healthier meals, exercising, or managing stress together, a support system makes it easier to stay consistent.

Online communities or local support groups can also offer advice, share experiences, and provide practical tips for living with gallbladder issues. Joining these groups allows you to connect with others who understand your journey, making it easier to stay motivated and informed about maintaining gallbladder health.

Balancing Work and Health

Balancing work with health priorities is key to maintaining a healthy lifestyle that supports gallbladder function. Schedule regular breaks for meals and avoid eating at your desk whenever possible, as taking time to eat mindfully can improve digestion. Plan your meals ahead and opt for healthy, fiber-rich foods that support gallbladder health to avoid the temptation of fast food during busy days.

Time management skills are also essential in balancing work and health. Set reminders to stretch, take brief walks, or practice deep breathing exercises throughout the day. Prioritizing these small actions can contribute to a healthier lifestyle that supports both your work efficiency and your gallbladder health.

Tips for Creating a Healthy Living Environment

Creating a healthy living environment can significantly impact gallbladder health by reducing stress and promoting better eating habits. Start by organizing your kitchen with nutritious foods, such as fresh fruits, vegetables, whole grains, and lean proteins. Minimize junk food and keep healthy snacks accessible to make better food choices easily.

Incorporate elements into your home that support relaxation and well-being, such as plants, natural light, or a designated area for meditation or stretching. By surrounding yourself with a supportive environment, you can cultivate habits that are beneficial to your gallbladder and overall health, making it easier to maintain a balanced lifestyle.

The Significance of Routine and Consistency

A consistent routine, including regular meal times and sleep schedules, is beneficial for gallbladder health as it helps regulate digestion and bile production. Plan your meals and avoid skipping them, as erratic eating can disrupt the digestive process and put strain on the gallbladder. Consistency helps your body develop a rhythm that supports optimal digestive function.

Developing a daily routine that includes exercise, stress management, and adequate sleep contributes to a balanced lifestyle that supports gallbladder health. Sticking to a routine also makes it easier to sustain healthy habits over time, which can reduce the risk of gallbladder disease and other digestive issues.

Using Technology to Track Health Habits

Technology can be a valuable tool in tracking health habits that support gallbladder function, such as meal tracking, exercise, and water intake. Apps for tracking food can help ensure you're consuming a balanced diet, while fitness trackers can monitor your physical activity levels. Keeping track of these habits can help you identify areas where you can improve to support your gallbladder.

Set reminders for taking breaks, drinking water, or doing stress-relief exercises throughout the day. Technology not only helps you stay accountable but also provides insights into patterns, making it easier to adjust your lifestyle and make informed decisions for better gallbladder health.

Engaging in Community Resources and Programs

Community resources, such as wellness programs, support groups, or local classes, can provide additional support for maintaining gallbladder health. Many communities offer group exercise sessions, nutrition workshops, or stress management classes, which can make adopting healthy habits more accessible and enjoyable. Check your local health centers or community centers for available programs.

Participating in these resources can offer a sense of camaraderie and accountability, making it easier to stay motivated in your health journey. Community programs also provide access to professional guidance, which can help you tailor lifestyle choices that are beneficial for gallbladder health and overall wellness.

Creating a Long-Term Health Plan

Creating a long-term health plan for gallbladder health involves setting realistic goals and outlining strategies for achieving them. Start by identifying areas you want to focus on, such as improving diet, increasing physical activity, or managing stress, and then break these goals into actionable steps. Review your progress periodically to adjust your plan as needed.

Incorporate elements that support sustainable habits, such as regular health check-ups, support networks, and community resources. A comprehensive plan ensures that you stay proactive about gallbladder health, reducing the likelihood of complications and helping you maintain an overall healthy lifestyle that supports your long-term wellness goals.

CHAPTER 8:

Surgical Interventions and Recovery

Overview of Surgical Options for Gallbladder Disease

Gallbladder disease is often treated with surgery, especially when gallstones cause pain or other complications. The most common surgical option is a cholecystectomy, which is the removal of the gallbladder. This procedure can be performed laparoscopically, which involves small incisions, or through open surgery for more complicated cases. Laparoscopic surgery is usually preferred because it is minimally invasive and has a shorter recovery time.

In addition to cholecystectomy, other surgical options include endoscopic retrograde cholangiopancreatography (ERCP) for removing stones from the bile duct, which can sometimes prevent the need for full gallbladder removal. Surgeons will assess the best option based on the severity of symptoms, the presence of infection, and the patient's overall health. Understanding the different procedures can help you make an informed decision with your healthcare provider.

What to Expect Before, During, and After Surgery

Before surgery, your healthcare provider will conduct tests, such as blood work and imaging scans, to ensure you're a good candidate. They'll also provide instructions on pre-operative care, which may include fasting and avoiding certain medications. During the procedure, you'll be under anesthesia, and the surgery typically takes about one to two hours, depending on whether it's laparoscopic or open.

After surgery, you'll be monitored in a recovery room until the anesthesia wears off. If you've had laparoscopic surgery, you can often go home the same day, while open surgery may require a few days in the hospital. You may experience some abdominal discomfort and bloating initially, but your medical team will guide you through managing these symptoms at home.

Importance of Pre-Operative Assessments

Pre-operative assessments are crucial for identifying any potential risks before surgery. These assessments typically include a physical exam, blood tests, and an ultrasound or MRI to confirm the presence and location of gallstones. If you have any underlying health issues, your doctor might recommend additional tests, such as an EKG or chest X-ray, to ensure that your heart and lungs can handle anesthesia.

These assessments help the surgical team prepare for any specific needs you may have during the procedure. For instance, if blood work reveals low platelet levels, they might adjust the surgical plan to reduce the risk of bleeding. A thorough pre-operative assessment not only improves safety but also aids in a smoother recovery.

Recovery Timeline and Milestones

The recovery timeline after gallbladder surgery varies depending on whether the surgery was laparoscopic or open. For laparoscopic surgery, many patients can return to light activities within a week and resume normal activities within two to four weeks. In contrast, open surgery may require a recovery period of six to eight weeks, with gradual increases in physical activity as the incisions heal.

Milestones during recovery include managing pain effectively, getting up and moving around to prevent blood clots, and gradually reintroducing solid foods.

By the third or fourth week, most laparoscopic surgery patients find they can return to regular routines, while open surgery patients will still need to take it easy to allow for proper healing.

Managing Pain Post-Surgery

Pain management is an important part of recovery after gallbladder surgery. Right after the surgery, you may experience soreness around the incision sites or in the shoulder area due to the gas used in laparoscopic procedures. Your doctor will likely prescribe pain medication for the first few days, which can then be tapered off as you start to feel better.

To manage pain effectively, it's recommended to avoid heavy lifting, take short walks to improve circulation, and apply heat packs to relieve muscle discomfort. Non-prescription options like acetaminophen or ibuprofen are usually sufficient for most patients as the pain subsides over the next few weeks.

Signs of Complications After Surgery

Knowing the signs of potential complications can help ensure a quick response if something goes wrong after gallbladder surgery. Common signs of complications include fever, severe pain, excessive redness or swelling at the incision sites, and difficulty breathing. You may also experience unusual symptoms like jaundice, which can indicate a bile duct injury.

If any of these symptoms occur, contact your healthcare provider immediately. Most complications are rare, especially with laparoscopic surgery, but prompt medical attention is important to address issues like infections or bile leaks that could require further treatment.

Role of Physical Therapy in Recovery

While not always necessary, physical therapy can be beneficial for patients who undergo open gallbladder surgery or experience post-operative complications. Physical therapy focuses on gentle exercises to improve core strength, reduce abdominal pain, and enhance mobility. Your therapist might also teach you breathing exercises to reduce discomfort from any residual abdominal gas.

These exercises can improve circulation and prevent stiffness, making it easier to return to normal activities over time. For some patients, physical therapy also helps to manage scar tissue, ensuring the incision area heals smoothly and restoring full movement to the abdomen.

Nutritional Needs During Recovery

Proper nutrition plays a significant role in recovery after gallbladder surgery. In the first few days, you'll likely follow a liquid diet and gradually reintroduce bland, low-fat foods. Foods rich in fiber and low in fat are easier on your digestive system and help reduce the risk of diarrhea, a common issue post-surgery.

As you progress, incorporate lean proteins, whole grains, and fruits and vegetables to support healing. Avoiding spicy and fatty foods helps prevent digestive discomfort. Staying hydrated and eating smaller, more frequent meals can also make digestion easier as your body adjusts to functioning without a gallbladder.

Importance of Follow-Up Appointments

Follow-up appointments are essential to monitor your progress and ensure your recovery is on track. Typically scheduled a week or two after surgery, these appointments allow your surgeon to check your incisions, address any concerns, and adjust your pain management plan if necessary.

In addition, follow-up visits provide an opportunity to discuss any new symptoms or challenges you might be facing. Your doctor may also offer dietary advice and assess whether you're ready to resume certain activities. Regular check-ins help ensure a smooth recovery and provide reassurance that your healing process is progressing well.

Adjusting to Life Without a Gallbladder

After gallbladder removal, your body will adjust to digesting food differently since bile flows directly from your liver to the small intestine. Many people find they can eat most of their favorite foods again over time, but it's advisable to start with a low-fat diet and slowly reintroduce other foods as your digestive system adapts.

Some individuals may experience occasional digestive symptoms, such as bloating or diarrhea, but these often improve within a few months. Staying mindful of portion sizes, eating smaller meals, and limiting high-fat foods can help ease this transition and keep you comfortable.

Common Misconceptions About Gallbladder Removal

One common misconception about gallbladder removal is that it will severely limit your diet permanently. While you may need to make temporary adjustments to allow your body to adapt, most people can return to a normal diet within a few months. Another misconception is that the gallbladder is essential for digestion; however, the liver continues to produce bile even without the gallbladder.

Additionally, some worry that surgery will lead to long-term digestive issues. In reality, most people experience only minor adjustments and can live healthy lives post-surgery. Understanding these misconceptions can ease anxiety and help you focus on a smooth recovery.

Strategies for Returning to Daily Activities

When it comes to resuming daily activities after gallbladder surgery, it's essential to take things slow. Start with light activities like walking to help improve circulation and prevent blood clots. Avoid heavy lifting, bending, and strenuous exercise until you get the green light from your doctor, usually around four to six weeks for laparoscopic surgery and longer for open surgery.

Gradually work up to more strenuous tasks, such as household chores or exercise routines, as your body allows. Listening to your body's signals and not rushing the process will help you regain strength and energy, making it easier to return to your normal routine comfortably.

Long-Term Effects of Surgery on Health

Most people who have their gallbladder removed live healthy, normal lives without long-term effects. However, some may experience occasional digestive issues, such as gas or diarrhea, especially when consuming fatty foods. Your digestive system can adapt over time, and eating a balanced, low-fat diet often reduces these symptoms.

In rare cases, individuals may develop post-cholecystectomy syndrome, which involves chronic digestive discomfort. Working with a healthcare provider to adjust your diet or lifestyle can alleviate symptoms. For most, though, the benefits of surgery—such as relief from pain and infections—far outweigh any long-term effects.

CHAPTER 9:

Common Concerns and FAQs

What are Gallstones, and How are They Formed?

Gallstones are small, hardened deposits that form in the gallbladder due to imbalances in bile substances like cholesterol and bilirubin. When these substances build up, they can crystallize into stones of various sizes. Some people may develop just one, while others have multiple gallstones, which can range from tiny grains to larger stones. Gallstones often form without any noticeable symptoms, but when they block bile ducts, they can cause pain and discomfort.

Gallstones typically form due to a variety of factors, including genetics, obesity, and certain dietary habits like high-fat intake. While many gallstones are "silent" and don't require treatment, others may cause significant pain and complications if they obstruct bile flow. Diagnosis typically involves imaging tests such as ultrasound or CT scans. Treatment depends on the severity and may include lifestyle changes, medication, or surgical removal of the gallbladder if necessary.

How Can I Prevent Gallbladder Disease?

To help prevent gallbladder disease, maintaining a healthy diet is essential. Avoiding high-fat and high-cholesterol foods, while incorporating more fiber, can keep bile from becoming overly saturated, reducing the likelihood of gallstone formation. Regular exercise and maintaining a healthy weight can also lower your risk, as obesity is a significant factor in developing gallbladder disease. Eating small, frequent meals instead of large, heavy meals is also beneficial.

Staying hydrated and limiting alcohol consumption can further support gallbladder health. Some studies suggest that incorporating healthy fats, like those from fish or olive oil, may improve bile flow, reducing the chance of gallstone formation. Managing any chronic conditions, such as diabetes, is also important, as they can contribute to an increased risk of gallbladder issues.

What Are the Risks of Gallbladder Surgery?

Gallbladder surgery, or cholecystectomy, is generally safe but does carry some risks like any surgical procedure. Common risks include infections at the surgical site, bleeding, and adverse reactions to anesthesia. In rare cases, injury to nearby organs, such as the bile ducts or intestines, can occur. Some patients may also experience digestive issues post-surgery, as the body adjusts to the absence of the gallbladder.

To minimize risks, your surgeon will perform a thorough pre-operative assessment and use minimally invasive techniques whenever possible. Most people recover well and notice significant relief from symptoms once the gallbladder is removed. However, it's important to follow post-surgery guidelines closely, including dietary adjustments and activity restrictions, to aid in a smooth recovery.

Can Gallbladder Disease Be Managed Without Surgery?

Yes, mild gallbladder disease can sometimes be managed through non-surgical methods, especially if the gallstones are small and not causing severe symptoms. Dietary changes, like reducing fat intake, can help alleviate symptoms and prevent further stone formation. Medications, such as bile acids, can sometimes dissolve small cholesterol-based gallstones, though this approach can take months and is not always effective.

For those who prefer non-surgical options, natural therapies like regular exercise, a fiber-rich diet, and weight management can be beneficial in managing symptoms. It's important to work with a healthcare provider to monitor gallbladder health, as untreated gallstones can lead to complications. For severe cases, surgery may be the only effective treatment.

How Does Diet Impact Gallbladder Health?

Diet plays a major role in gallbladder health, as high-fat and high-cholesterol foods can lead to gallstone formation. A balanced diet rich in fruits, vegetables, lean proteins, and whole grains helps keep bile in a liquid state, reducing the risk of stones. Healthy fats from sources like fish, nuts, and olive oil are better choices than saturated fats, as they promote good bile flow.

Additionally, limiting refined carbohydrates and sugars can prevent bile imbalance and reduce inflammation, which helps maintain overall gallbladder health. Eating smaller, more frequent meals throughout the day can also prevent bile from building up, making digestion smoother and decreasing stress on the gallbladder.

What Symptoms Should Prompt a Doctor Visit?

If you experience severe abdominal pain, particularly on the right side under your rib cage, you should consult a doctor. Pain that radiates to the back or shoulder, nausea, vomiting, fever, and jaundice are all possible signs of gallbladder disease and should be addressed promptly. These symptoms may indicate a gallstone blockage or an infection, both of which require medical attention.

Additionally, persistent indigestion, bloating, or discomfort after eating fatty foods can also suggest gallbladder issues. Early diagnosis and treatment can prevent more serious complications, so it's essential to seek medical advice if you experience any unusual or severe symptoms.

Can Gallstones Cause Serious Complications?

Yes, untreated gallstones can lead to serious complications. If a gallstone blocks the bile duct, it can cause inflammation or infection of the gallbladder, known as cholecystitis. This condition can lead to intense pain, fever, and a risk of bursting, which is a medical emergency. Gallstones can also block the pancreatic duct, causing pancreatitis, a painful inflammation of the pancreas.

In severe cases, untreated gallstones may result in gangrene of the gallbladder or bile duct infections that can spread to the bloodstream, leading to sepsis. These complications are why it's crucial to monitor gallstones and seek treatment if symptoms worsen.

How Long Does Recovery from Gallbladder Surgery Take?

Recovery from gallbladder surgery, particularly when done laparoscopically, typically takes about one to two weeks for most people to return to normal activities. For the first few days, you may experience mild discomfort at the incision site, bloating, or fatigue, which gradually improves.

You'll likely need to avoid heavy lifting and intense physical activity during this initial recovery period.

It's essential to follow your doctor's post-operative instructions, including dietary changes, as the body adjusts to the absence of the gallbladder. For some, digestive changes may occur, so eating smaller, low-fat meals can ease the transition.

Are There Any Natural Remedies for Gallbladder Health?

Several natural remedies may support gallbladder health and prevent gallstone formation. For example, consuming a diet rich in fiber from fruits and vegetables can help with digestion and reduce bile cholesterol levels. Additionally, herbs like milk thistle and turmeric are often suggested for their anti-inflammatory properties, though more research is needed to confirm their effectiveness.

Incorporating healthy fats from sources like olive oil and fish may improve bile flow and prevent stone formation. Regular physical activity and weight management are also recommended to keep the gallbladder functioning optimally. While these remedies can be beneficial, they are not substitutes for medical treatment if you already have gallstones or gallbladder disease.

Can I Still Live a Normal Life After Gallbladder Removal?

Yes, most people live normal, healthy lives after gallbladder removal. Since the liver still produces bile, it flows directly into the small intestine, though in a less regulated way than before. This can lead to digestive changes, but these often improve with time and dietary adjustments. Avoiding large, fatty meals and focusing on smaller, balanced meals can help your body adjust.

Many individuals report improved quality of life after gallbladder removal due to the elimination of painful symptoms. While some people may experience mild digestive changes, such as diarrhea or bloating, these symptoms are usually manageable with dietary modifications and typically lessen over time.

How Often Should I See My Doctor After Treatment?

After gallbladder surgery, you'll likely have a follow-up appointment within a few weeks to ensure proper healing and recovery. For those managing gallbladder disease non-surgically, periodic check-ups, especially if you experience any new or worsening symptoms, can help prevent complications. Your doctor may recommend ultrasound or other imaging tests to monitor gallstones and gallbladder health.

If you're on medication or have other conditions, regular visits every six months to a year may be advisable. Staying proactive with follow-up care helps address any issues early, ensuring long-term gallbladder health and overall well-being.

What Lifestyle Changes Can I Make to Support My Gallbladder Health?

Maintaining a healthy diet low in fats and high in fiber can significantly benefit gallbladder health. Incorporate more fruits, vegetables, lean proteins, and whole grains into your meals, and avoid processed and high-cholesterol foods. Staying hydrated and limiting alcohol consumption can also support gallbladder function and reduce the risk of stone formation.

Exercise and maintaining a healthy weight are also important. Regular physical activity helps regulate digestion and lowers cholesterol, which reduces the risk of gallstones. Making these lifestyle changes not only supports gallbladder health but also contributes to overall physical wellness.

Where Can I Find Support and Resources for Gallbladder Disease?

Many resources are available to help you manage gallbladder disease. Support groups, both online and in-person, provide a space to share experiences and tips with others who understand your situation. Websites like the American Liver Foundation and the National Institute of Diabetes and Digestive and Kidney Diseases offer valuable information on gallbladder health, treatment options, and lifestyle advice.

Consulting a dietitian can also provide guidance on meal planning to support your gallbladder health. Talking to your healthcare provider about local resources and support groups can help you stay informed and connected with others going through similar experiences.

Conclusion

Understanding gallbladder disease and its implications is crucial for managing health effectively. With appropriate dietary adjustments, lifestyle changes, and medical interventions, individuals can navigate their journey toward improved gallbladder health.

Awareness of symptoms, regular check-ups, and education about treatment options empower individuals to take control of their health and make informed decisions about their well-being. Seeking guidance from healthcare professionals, utilizing community resources, and connecting with support groups can further enhance the management of gallbladder disease. By prioritizing gallbladder health, individuals can lead fulfilling lives with reduced risk of complications.

www.ingramcontent.com/pod-product-compliance
Lightning Source LLC
Chambersburg PA
CBHW071511220526
45472CB00003B/983